PRITIKIN DIET
&
MEAL PLAN
COOKBOOK

Recipes and Meal Plans for Weight Loss and Optimal Health: Delicious Recipes for Every Day

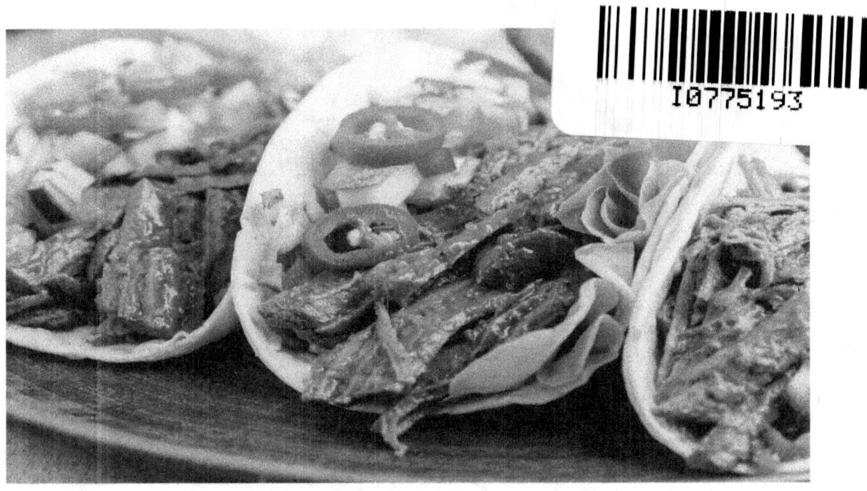

OLIVIA MITCHELL

Table of Contents

COPYRIGHT

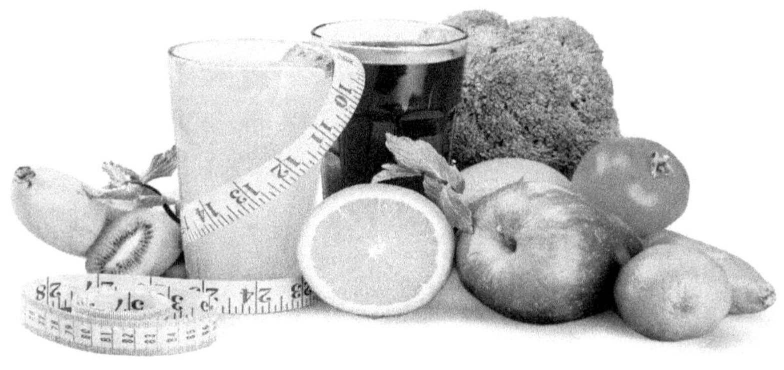

 Pritkin Diet and Meal Plan

INTRODUCTION

Picture a place with all those wonderful meals comprised of taste, nutrition, and joy. Vibrant colors which playfully leap off your plate onto your taste buds but always care for your health. That is the world that will welcome you in this same book that you are about to open.

Tosh this diet cook book. These are not boring, flavorless foods made to ruin your taste buds! This is an explosive gastronomic upheavals, a festivity of tastes that simultaneously stimulate the palate and give health benefits.

Have a look at these beautiful pictures of delicious and colorful salads. Can't imagine hearty soups simmering on your stove, full of warmth and nutrition waiting for you? Imagine indulging with the luscious tastes of main courses tickling your palate; every mouthful a confirmation that great tasting and healthy can indeed go together.

However, this voyage involves more than just food. The recipes are carefully made and follow the old proven principles for Pritikin. Every ingredient specially selected will form a brick for your wellness, giving you necessary vitamins that drive your organism and spirit.

Now, recall the latest purchase of a cookbook that you did. Did it inspire you and make you feel strong enough to try out new recipes? Was it an actual guide to good living or simply a cook book?

The friend, this book is unlike any other. Your road map to a healthy delicious world. Are reservoir of knowledge for information about the Pritikin diet and how healthy eating can become part of your daily life.

Therefore, flip the page and embark on the exciting journey of cooking. Unravel the mysteries of turning healthy food into songs to your soul. The power of healthy eating and loving every bite.

It is not just a cookbook but rather the key to a healthy and happy LIFE . Accept such mysteries, and it will become clear to you very shortly that such a simple thing as a cookbook is in fact your constant friend on the way of health perfection.

CHAPTER 1

THE PRITIKIN DIET: A Comprehensive Guide

A NEW HEALTH AND WELLNESS CULTURE

Starting on a new diet can be so scary. You get a lot of contradictions and numerous options to choose from. However, the Pritikin diet is a different case entirely. It's not just a band-aid; it's an entire healthy living programme that empowers you to take control of your health long-term. This chapter will be your guide, helping you understand the key elements of the Pritikin Diet so that you can start with the right foot on this journey of transformation.

UNDERSTANDING THE CORE PHILOSOPHY OF PRITIKIN DIET

The Pritikin Diet is based on a deep understanding of the link between food and lifestyle. In the seventies it was developed as a low-fat, high-fiber based plant nutritious approach by the visionary Dr. Nathan Pritikin. The dietary philosophy of this diet goes beyond simple calorie restriction; it entails eating whole, unprocessed foods that feed and provide the body with vitamins, minerals, and fibre.

THE POWER OF PLANT-BASED EATING

The basis of the Pritikin diet comprises fruits, vegetables, whole grain, legumes, nuts, and seeds. These plant based powerhouses are loaded with nutrients that give you energy, cleanse your system, make you feel good, among others. You'll, therefore, consume healthy foods, with low content of unhealthy fats, cholesterol, and sodium, known to cause ailments such as heart disease, stroke, diabetes, among others.

BEYOND THE PLATE: Embracing a Holistic Lifestyle

The Pritikin, however, does not stop at merely eating. Exercise is one of its focus areas because it highlights the role it plays in keeping heart healthy, controlling weight, and enhancing mood. The program includes regular personal exercise that suits your personal taste or desires. Besides, inner strength could be achieved through practicing such stress management techniques as yoga or meditations which further contribute to one's general health.

TAKING THE FIRST STEP: Embracing Change

A new diet can always seem intimidating but does not have to. The Pritikin Program provides you with all the tools and resources you need to succeed, including:

Comprehensive meal plans and recipes: Discover a wealth of delicacies and fresh meals that are easy to plan for and cook.

- **Support and guidance:** Become part of a network of similar people, with a supportive professional help provided by Pritikin Program's experts.

- **Educational resources:** Find out everything about Pritikin diet science, as well as nutrition basics for a proper lifestyle.

- Pritikin Diet means more than changing diets but lifetime commitment. If you embrace those of its' principles, your path to a healthier, happier, meaningful future will start.

Are you willing to be in charge of your health? Flip the page and venture further into the realm of the Pritikin Diet. Equipping you with the necessary information and tools to unleash your true power is what we strive for—a life that will truly be an adventure!

THE BENEFITS OF THE PRITIKIN DIET

UNLOCKING A HEALTHIER, HAPPIER YOU

Pritikin Diet is not your everyday diet. It is much more than that; it is a lifestyle that changes one's life completely, opening up new possibilities for health and happiness. It is a lot greater than simply adding to the scale of your life; it will touch many things in your life that perhaps you don't understand. Let's delve into the world-changing effects of the Pritkin Diet, its benefits on every level of your being.

1. Lose Weight Permanently and Get a New Look.

Pritikin Diet disrupts the phenomenon of yo-yo dieting. This emphasizes on whole, non-processed plant-based food, naturally leading to weight loss without return. Eating less unhealthy fats and refined carbohydrates will mean feeling fuller for extended periods thereby avoiding constant snacking and restrictive diet plans that count calories. Losing weight through practicing the Pritikin way is an ongoing exercise, making one consume healthily as a natural habit.

2. Minimize the risk of chronic diseases and support optimum health.

The Pritikin Diet is not only for losing weight, but also for preventing diseases. Research indicates that following this dietary pattern substantially cuts down on developing chronic conditions such as cardiovascular ailments, stroke, diabetes, and even certain forms of cancers. This is achieved through several mechanisms, including:

- Improves the cholesterol level as well as controls high blood pressures.
- Reducing inflammation
- Improving blood sugar control

- Promoting gut health

The Pritikin diet is an investment into your future good health and protection against related health risks along the way to a long and happy life.

3. Spark an onslaught of energy and vitality.

Do you feel tired all the time? Have you heard of Pritikin Diet? You will naturally gain more energy when you feed your body on wholesome, nutrition rich foods. The newly-founded energy can also transform into enhanced production rates, higher level of performance in sports and an added zeal for life. Leave behind the late afternoon sleepiness and welcome heightened vigor with the Pritikin way.

4. Lift Your Spirits and Find Serenity Inside.

Your gut and your brain are powerfully linked according to the Pritikin Diet. Feeding your gut micro-biome good bacteria found in whole plant-based foods leads to production of happiness inducing neuro transmitters such as serotonin. This can lead to:

- Improved mood
- Reduced stress levels
- Enhanced mental clarity
- Increased resilience
- Better sleep quality

The Pritikin diet is not only about physical health but also involves mental relaxation as one strives for happiness in all other areas.

5. Enjoy a world of tasty and nutritious food.

Living on Pritikin Diet does not necessarily equate to a monotonous diet with bland food restrictions. On the contrary, it serves as an opening for a new world of scrumptious, healthy food. Do not worry, you will be amazed at the number of meals you'll make using whole grains, legumes, fruits, vegetables, and nuts. Pritikin Program has a ton of mouthwatering recipes that will feed both your taste buds and your body.

Live vibrantly, embrace total health.

Actually, Pritikin diet is not only a diet but also an investment towards the future. Embracing those principles is an investment in life full of vitality, robust energy, and optimism. Note that you are not embarking on this exodus alone. They offer support to you while on your journey in their Pritikin program.

Are you set for Pritikin transformation? Turn the page and start your way to healthier, happy, and satisfactory you.

HOW TO USE THIS COOKBOOK

YOUR ROADMAP TO SUCCESS

Welcome aboard, and good luck for starting Pritikin diet on your way to a better you. The cookbook acts as your personal guide through the program to access its transformative elements. Here's how to maximize your experience and make the most of this valuable resource:

1. Familiarize Yourself with the Pritikin Principles:

However, it is important to familiarize yourself with the basics of the Pritikin Diet before jumping straight into its recipes. This includes:

The importance of whole, unprocessed foods: These should include fruits, vegetables, whole grains, beans, nuts, and seeds.

Limiting unhealthy fats: Make sure to use healthy fats like in avocadoes, nuts, seeds and minimize the intake of saturated and trans fats.

Choosing lean protein sources: Consider having fish, chicken, or beans as sources of lean protein in moderation.

Minimizing refined carbohydrates: Go for minimal sodas, processed snacks and white breads.

Making exercise a priority: Adhere to moderate levels of exercise that is suitable for you.

Having a good grasp of these fundamentals will enable you to choose intelligently when it comes to adjusting recipes to suit your tastes.

2. Explore the Chapters and Find Inspiration:

This is a cookbook for you that offers all kinds of tasty Pritikin diet recipes. Explore the various chapters:

Breakfast: Find out about wholesome and strong choices that will keep you going throughout the day.

Lunch: Opt for light and filling dishes for lunch.

Dinner: Find a range of tasty and exciting dinners.

Snacks: Find nutritious and easy-to-carry snack bars for those on-the-go moments during long working hours.

Desserts: Satisfy your taste buds and get away with sinful Pritikin-compliant desserts.

Side Dishes: Make sure that you serve tasty and nutritious side dishes on your main meals.

Sauces and Dips: Make flavored homemade sauces and dips for elevating your cooking.

Meal Planning: Find helpful suggestions for meal planning, keeping to your budget and achieving success.

Resources: Find more information on Pritikin Diet and how to lead a healthy life.

3. Utilize the Recipe Features:

Each recipe offers valuable information to guide you through the cooking process:

Ingredients: The listed ingredients will clearly indicate all you expect in the pack before using it.

Instructions: Guided step-by-step ensures that even an inexperienced cook can successfully produce the desired outcome.

Nutrition Information: Get the servings size and check the nutrition facts for each serving such as; amount of calories, total fats, proteins, carbohydrate, dietary fibre, and sodium.

Tips and Variations: Find out ideas and changes that can be undertaken to suit your tastes or custom diet requirements.

4. Make it Your Own:

A cookbook for you, with recipes that are not set in stone. Do not hesitate to try out new recipes, replace what you do not like with whatever you prefer, and discover different methods of cooking.

Ensure you remember that while on the Pritikin diet you are allowed to modify it based on what suits you well.

5. Join the Community:

Sharing your goals towards health and fitness makes the whole journey fun and worthwhile. You can also join the Pritikin community by participating in the online forums and various social media groups as well as the local support groups. Share your experience, get motivate and study other's experiences while journeying.

Unlocking a Healthier Future:

Indeed, The Pritikin diet can be a very useful instrument for turning around your life. This cookbook will be your companion as you discover a galaxy of healthy, delectable food products. Keep in mind that the process will be as rewarding as reaching your goal at the end of it all…. Enjoy the process, discover new tastes, and celebrate your milestones as you proceed. With determination and backup, in front of you there is a more joyous and vigorous future.

CHAPTER 2

BREAKFAST:

Delicious and Nutritious Pritikin Breakfasts

Rise and shine to a new day brimming with energy and vitality! Breakfast is the cornerstone of a healthy Pritikin lifestyle, setting the tone for your entire day. Forget the sugary cereals and greasy pastries – this chapter unveils a treasure trove of delicious and nutritious breakfast recipes that will tantalize your taste buds and fuel your body for optimal performance.

Here are 10 breakfast recipes to jumpstart your mornings:

1. Spiced Oatmeal with Berries and Nuts

Ingredients:

- 1/2 cup rolled oats
- 1 cup unsweetened plant-based milk
- 1/4 cup water
- 1/4 teaspoon cinnamon
- 1/8 teaspoon ginger
- Pinch of salt

- 1/4 cup fresh berries

- 2 tablespoons chopped nuts

- Maple syrup or honey (optional)

Instructions:

- Combine rolled oats, plant-based milk, water, cinnamon, ginger, and salt in a saucepan.

- Bring to a simmer over medium heat, stirring occasionally.

- Reduce heat and cook for 5-7 minutes, stirring occasionally, until oats are tender.

- Divide oatmeal into bowls and top with berries, nuts, and maple syrup or honey (optional).

2. **Scrumptious Tofu Scramble**

Ingredients:

- 14 ounces firm tofu, drained and crumbled

- 1 tablespoon olive oil

- 1/2 onion, chopped

- 1 bell pepper, chopped

- 1 cup spinach, chopped

- 1/2 teaspoon turmeric

- 1/4 teaspoon black salt

- 1/4 cup nutritional yeast

- Whole-wheat toast or whole-grain tortillas

Instructions:

- In a skillet, heat olive oil over medium heat.
- Add onion and cook until softened, about 5 minutes.
- Add bell pepper and cook for 3 minutes more.
- Add spinach and cook until wilted.
- Add crumbled tofu, turmeric, black salt, and nutritional yeast.
- Cook for 5 minutes, stirring occasionally, until heated through.
- Serve tofu scramble on toast or tortillas.

3. **Power-Packed Smoothie Bowl**

Ingredients:

- 1 banana, frozen
- 1 cup fresh berries
- 1 cup spinach
- 1 cup unsweetened plant-based milk
- 1 scoop protein powder
- Granola, chia seeds, or chopped nuts (optional)
- Instructions:
- Blend all ingredients in a blender until smooth and creamy.

- Pour the smoothie into a bowl and top with desired toppings.

4. Overnight Oats with Chia Seeds and Fruit

Ingredients:

- 1/2 cup rolled oats
- 1 tablespoon chia seeds
- 1/2 cup unsweetened plant-based milk
- 1/4 cup yogurt
- 1/4 cup chopped fruit

Instructions:

- Layer rolled oats, chia seeds, plant-based milk, yogurt, and chopped fruit in a jar.
- Seal the jar and refrigerate overnight.
- In the morning, give the oats a stir and enjoy them cold or warmed up.

5. Whole-Wheat Pancakes with Berries and Yogurt

Ingredients:

- 1 cup whole-wheat flour
- 1 tablespoon baking powder

- 1/4 teaspoon salt

- 1/2 teaspoon cinnamon

- 1 1/4 cups unsweetened plant-based milk

- 1/4 cup yogurt

- 1 egg (or flaxseed egg)

- Fresh berries

- Nonfat Greek yogurt

Instructions:

- In a bowl, whisk together flour, baking powder, salt, and cinnamon.

- In another bowl, whisk together plant-based milk, yogurt, and egg (or flaxseed egg).

- Add the wet ingredients to the dry ingredients and whisk until just combined.

- Heat a lightly greased griddle or pan over medium heat.

- Pour 1/4 cup batter onto the griddle for each pancake.

- Cook for 2-3 minutes per side, or until golden brown.

- Serve pancakes with fresh berries and nonfat Greek yogurt.

6. Savory Quinoa Breakfast Bowl

Ingredients:

- 1 cup quinoa, cooked

- 1 tablespoon olive oil
- 1/2 onion, chopped
- 1 cup mushrooms, chopped
- 1 cup spinach, chopped
- 1/2 cup tomatoes, chopped
- Herbs and spices to taste

Instructions:

- Cook quinoa according to package instructions.
- In a skillet, heat olive oil over medium heat.
- Add onion and cook until softened, about 5 minutes.
- Add mushrooms and cook for 5 minutes more.
- Add spinach and cook until wilted.
- Add tomatoes and cook for 2 minutes more.
- Combine cooked quinoa with sautéed

7. Whole-Wheat Toast with Avocado and Egg

Ingredients:

- 2 slices whole-wheat bread
- 1 ripe avocado, mashed
- 1 egg (poached or fried)
- Salt and pepper to taste

Instructions:

- Toast whole-wheat bread to desired level of crispness.

- Spread mashed avocado on toast.

- Top with a poached or fried egg.

- Season with salt and pepper to taste.

8. Chia Pudding with Berries and Coconut

Ingredients:

- 1/4 cup chia seeds

- 1 cup unsweetened plant-based milk

- 1/4 cup coconut milk

- 1/4 cup fresh berries

- 1 tablespoon shredded coconut

Instructions:

- Combine chia seeds, plant-based milk, and coconut milk in a jar.

- Stir well and refrigerate for at least 4 hours, or overnight for a thicker consistency.

- In the morning, top the pudding with fresh berries and shredded coconut.

9. Smoothie with Protein Powder and Greens

Ingredients:

- 1 frozen banana

- 1 cup spinach

- 1 scoop protein powder

- 1 cup unsweetened plant-based milk

- 1/4 cup fresh or frozen berries (optional)

Instructions:

- Combine all ingredients in a blender.

- Blend until smooth and creamy.

- Enjoy immediately or pour into a travel container for a grab-and-go breakfast.

10. Baked Oatmeal with Apples and Pecans

Ingredients:

- 1/2 cup rolled oats

- 1/2 cup unsweetened plant-based milk

- 1/4 cup water

- 1/4 cup chopped apple

- 1/4 cup chopped pecans

- 1/4 teaspoon cinnamon

- 1/4 teaspoon nutmeg

- 1/4 cup unsweetened applesauce

- Maple syrup or honey (optional)

Instructions:

- Preheat oven to 375°F (190°C).

- Combine rolled oats, plant-based milk, water, chopped apple, pecans, cinnamon, nutmeg, and applesauce in a baking dish.

- Bake for 25-30 minutes, or until golden brown and bubbly.

- Serve warm with maple syrup or honey (optional).

These 10 delicious and nutritious Pritikin breakfast recipes offer a variety of flavors and textures to keep your mornings exciting and satisfying. Remember, breakfast is the most important meal of the day, so start yours off right with a Pritikin-approved meal that fuels your body and sets the tone for a healthy and vibrant day.

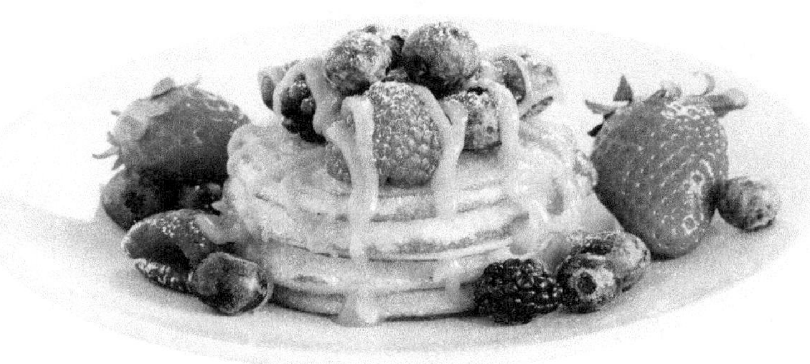

CHAPTER 3

LUNCH:

Light and Nutritious Pritikin Lunches

Say goodbye to the midday slump! Chapter 3 is your guide to creating delicious and energizing Pritikin-approved lunches that fuel your body and keep you focused throughout the afternoon. No more settling for unhealthy, greasy options – these recipes are packed with flavor and nutrients, leaving you feeling satisfied and ready to conquer the rest of your day.

Here are 10 nutritious and satisfying Pritikin lunch recipes:

1. Rainbow Veggie Wraps with Hummus

Ingredients:

- 2 whole-wheat tortillas
- 1/2 cup hummus
- 1/2 cup bell peppers, chopped (assorted colors)
- 1/2 cup carrots, chopped
- 1/2 cup cucumbers, chopped
- 2 cups spinach
- 1/2 cup sprouts

- 1 avocado, sliced (optional)

Instructions:

- Spread hummus evenly on each tortilla.
- Layer bell peppers, carrots, cucumbers, and spinach on each tortilla.
- Top with sprouts and avocado slices (optional).
- Roll up the tortillas tightly and enjoy!

2. **Lentil Soup with Whole-Wheat Bread**

Ingredients:

- 1 tablespoon olive oil
- 1 onion, chopped
- 2 carrots, chopped
- 2 celery stalks, chopped
- 4 cups vegetable broth
- 1 cup lentils, rinsed
- 1 teaspoon cumin
- 1/2 teaspoon turmeric
- Salt and pepper to taste
- 4 slices whole-wheat bread

Instructions:

- Heat olive oil in a large pot over medium heat.
- Add onion, carrots, and celery, and cook until softened, about 5 minutes.
- Add vegetable broth, lentils, cumin, and turmeric. Bring to a boil, then reduce heat and simmer for 30 minutes, or until lentils are tender.
- Season with salt and pepper to taste.
- Serve hot with whole-wheat bread.

3. **Quinoa Salad with Roasted Vegetables and Herbs**

Ingredients:

- 1 cup quinoa, rinsed
- 1 tablespoon olive oil
- 1/2 teaspoon cumin
- 1/2 teaspoon paprika
- 1 sweet potato, chopped
- 1 zucchini, chopped
- 1 red onion, chopped
- 1/4 cup chopped fresh parsley
- 1/4 cup chopped fresh cilantro
- Vinaigrette dressing (your favorite)

Instructions:

- Preheat oven to 400°F (200°C).
- Toss sweet potato, zucchini, and onion with olive oil, cumin, and paprika.
- Spread vegetables on a baking sheet and roast for 20-25 minutes, or until tender.
- Cook quinoa according to package instructions.
- Combine cooked quinoa, roasted vegetables, parsley, and cilantro.
- Drizzle with vinaigrette dressing and toss to coat.
- Serve chilled or at room temperature.

4. **Turkey and Veggie Lettuce Wraps**

Ingredients:

- 1 pound ground turkey
- 1 onion, chopped
- 2 cloves garlic, minced
- 1 teaspoon paprika
- 1/2 teaspoon chili powder
- 4 large lettuce leaves
- 1 carrot, shredded
- 1 avocado, sliced

- Yogurt-based sauce (your favorite)

Instructions:

- Brown ground turkey in a large skillet over medium heat.
- Add onion and garlic, and cook until softened, about 5 minutes.
- Stir in paprika and chili powder.
- Spoon cooked turkey mixture into lettuce leaves.
- Top with shredded carrots, avocado slices, and yogurt-based sauce.
- Serve immediately.

5. **Black Bean Burgers with Sweet Potato Fries**

Ingredients:

- 1 (15-ounce) can black beans, drained and rinsed
- 1/2 cup cooked oats
- 1/4 cup breadcrumbs
- 1 teaspoon cumin
- 1/2 teaspoon chili powder
- 1/4 cup chopped fresh cilantro
- 1 tablespoon olive oil
- 1 sweet potato, peeled and cut into fries
- Paprika (optional)

     Pritkin Diet and Meal Plan

- Garlic powder (optional)
- Whole-wheat buns
- Hamburger toppings (lettuce, tomato, avocado)

Instructions:

- Mash black beans in a large bowl.
- Add oats, breadcrumbs, cumin, chili powder, and cilantro. Mix well.
- Form mixture into 4 patties.
- Heat olive oil in a skillet over medium heat.
- Add black bean burgers and cook for 5-7 minutes per side, or until golden brown.
- Meanwhile, preheat oven to 400°F (200°C).
- Toss sweet potato fries with olive oil, paprika (optional), and garlic powder (optional).
- Spread fries on a baking sheet and bake for 20-25 minutes, or until crisp.
- Serve black bean burgers on whole-wheat buns with desired toppings.

6. **Edamame Salad with Brown Rice and Sesame Ginger Dressing**

Ingredients:

- 1 cup brown rice, cooked
- 1 cup edamame pods, steamed or boiled
- 1/2 cup cucumber, chopped
- 1/2 cup carrots, chopped
- 1/4 cup crumbled tofu (optional)
- Sesame ginger dressing (your favorite)
- Sesame seeds

Instructions:

- Combine cooked brown rice, edamame pods, cucumber, carrots, and tofu (optional) in a large bowl.
- Drizzle with sesame ginger dressing and toss to coat.
- Garnish with sesame seeds and serve.

7. **Tuna Salad with Celery and Apples on Whole-Wheat Crackers**

Ingredients:

- 1 (5-ounce) can tuna packed in water, drained
- 1/4 cup celery, chopped
- 1/4 cup apple, chopped
- 1 tablespoon lemon juice
- Salt and pepper to taste
- Whole-wheat crackers

Instructions:

- Flake tuna in a bowl.
- Add chopped celery, apple, and lemon juice.
- Season with salt and pepper to taste.
- Serve on whole-wheat crackers.

8. **Greek Yogurt Parfait with Berries and Granola**

Ingredients:

- 1 cup plain Greek yogurt
- 1/2 cup granola
- 1/2 cup fresh berries (your favorite)
- Honey or maple syrup (optional)
- Instructions:
- Layer Greek yogurt, granola, and berries in a glass or jar.
- Drizzle with honey or maple syrup (optional).
- Serve immediately.

9. **Leftover Salmon Salad with Whole-Wheat Toast**

Ingredients:

 Pritkin Diet and Meal Plan

- 1 cup leftover cooked salmon, flaked
- 1/4 cup celery, chopped
- 1/4 cup red onion, chopped
- 1 tablespoon chopped fresh dill
- 1/2 cup plain Greek yogurt
- Salt and pepper to taste
- 2 slices whole-wheat bread, toasted
- Fresh dill sprigs (optional)
- Lemon wedge (optional)

Instructions:

- Combine flaked salmon, celery, red onion, and dill in a bowl.
- Stir in Greek yogurt and season with salt and pepper to taste.
- Spread salmon salad on toasted whole-wheat bread.
- Garnish with fresh dill sprigs and a lemon wedge (optional).

10. Chicken Caesar Salad with Light Dressing

Ingredients:

- 1 grilled or baked chicken breast, sliced
- 2 cups romaine lettuce, chopped

- 1/4 cup light Caesar dressing

- Shaved Parmesan cheese

- Croutons

- Fresh lemon juice

- Black pepper

Instructions:

- Arrange romaine lettuce on a plate.

- Top with sliced chicken breast, Parmesan cheese, and croutons.

- Drizzle with light Caesar dressing.

- Squeeze fresh lemon juice over the salad.

- Season with black pepper to taste.

- Serve immediately.

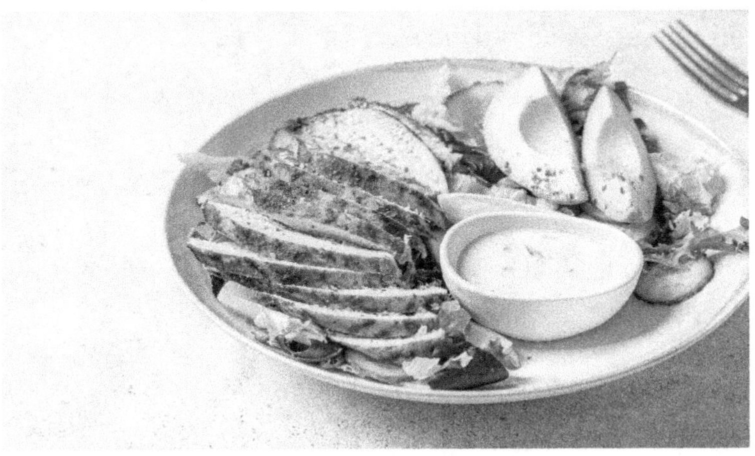

CHAPTER 4

DINNER:

Delicious and Nutritious Pritikin Dinners

As the day winds down and the sun sets, it's time to gather around the table and nourish your body with a satisfying and healthy dinner. Chapter 4 presents a delightful collection of Pritikin-approved recipes that are not only delicious but also fuel your body for a restful night and a vibrant tomorrow. From vibrant roasted vegetables to flavorful stir-fries, hearty lentil tacos to comforting vegetarian chili, and a classic spaghetti with whole-wheat twist, these recipes offer something for every palate and dietary preference. Let's dive into some culinary treats that will leave you feeling energized and satisfied.

1. **Salmon with Roasted Vegetables:**

Ingredients:

- 2 salmon fillets
- 1 tablespoon olive oil
- 1/2 teaspoon dried oregano
- 1/4 teaspoon salt
- 1/4 teaspoon black pepper

- 1 cup broccoli florets
- 1/2 cup red bell pepper, sliced
- 1/2 cup yellow bell pepper, sliced
- 1/2 cup red onion, sliced

Instructions:

- Preheat oven to 400°F (200°C).
- In a bowl, toss salmon with olive oil, oregano, salt, and pepper.
- Arrange salmon on a baking sheet lined with parchment paper.
- Toss broccoli, bell peppers, and onion with olive oil, salt, and pepper.
- Spread vegetables around the salmon on the baking sheet.
- Bake for 20-25 minutes, or until salmon is cooked through and vegetables are tender.

2. **Chicken Stir-Fry with Brown Rice:**

Ingredients:

- 1 pound boneless, skinless chicken breasts, cut into thin strips
- 1 tablespoon olive oil
- 1 onion, chopped

 Pritkin Diet and Meal Plan

- 2 cloves garlic, minced
- 1 cup broccoli florets
- 1 cup red bell pepper, sliced
- 1 cup yellow bell pepper, sliced
- 1/2 cup baby carrots
- 1/4 cup soy sauce
- 1 tablespoon cornstarch
- 1 cup cooked brown rice

Instructions:

- In a bowl, combine soy sauce and cornstarch to make a slurry.
- Heat olive oil in a large skillet or wok over medium-high heat.
- Add chicken and cook until browned, about 5 minutes.
- Add onion and garlic, and cook until softened, about 3 minutes.
- Add broccoli, bell peppers, and carrots, and cook for 5 minutes.
- Stir in the soy sauce mixture and cook until thickened, about 1 minute.
- Serve over cooked brown rice.

 Pritkin Diet and Meal Plan

3. Lentil Tacos:

Ingredients:

- 1 cup lentils, rinsed
- 1 cup vegetable broth
- 1/2 cup chopped onion
- 1/4 cup chopped celery
- 2 cloves garlic, minced
- 1 teaspoon cumin
- 1/2 teaspoon chili powder
- 1/4 teaspoon smoked paprika
- 1/4 cup chopped fresh cilantro
- 1/4 cup salsa
- 4 whole-wheat tortillas
- Avocado slices (optional)
- Lime wedges (optional)

Instructions:

- In a medium saucepan, combine lentils, vegetable broth, onion, celery, garlic, cumin, chili powder, and paprika.
- Bring to a boil, then reduce heat and simmer for 20-30 minutes, or until lentils are tender.
- Stir in cilantro and salsa.
- Warm tortillas according to package instructions.

- Fill tortillas with lentil mixture.

- Top with avocado slices and lime wedges (optional).

4. Vegetarian Chili:

Ingredients:

- 1 tablespoon olive oil

- 1 onion, chopped

- 2 carrots, chopped

- 2 celery stalks, chopped

- 2 cloves garlic, minced

- 1 (15-ounce) can kidney beans, drained and rinsed

- 1 (15-ounce) can black beans, drained and rinsed

- 1 (14.5-ounce) can diced tomatoes, undrained

- 1 cup vegetable broth

- 1 tablespoon chili powder

- 1 teaspoon cumin

- 1/2 teaspoon smoked paprika

- 1/4 teaspoon salt

- 1/4 teaspoon black pepper

Instructions:

- Heat olive oil in a large pot or Dutch oven over medium heat.

 Pritkin Diet and Meal Plan

- Add onion, carrots, and celery, and cook until softened, about 5 minutes.
- Add garlic and cook for 1 minute.
- Stir in kidney beans, black beans, tomatoes with their juices, vegetable broth, chili powder, cumin, paprika

5. **Spaghetti with Whole-Wheat Pasta and Tomato Sauce:**

Ingredients:

- 1 pound whole-wheat spaghetti
- 1 tablespoon olive oil
- 1 onion, chopped
- 2 cloves garlic, minced
- 1 (28-ounce) can crushed tomatoes
- 1 tablespoon tomato paste
- 1 teaspoon dried oregano
- 1/2 teaspoon dried basil
- 1/4 cup chopped fresh parsley
- Salt and pepper to taste

Instructions:

- Cook spaghetti according to package instructions.

                    Pritkin Diet and Meal Plan

- Meanwhile, heat olive oil in a large skillet over medium heat.
- Add onion and garlic, and cook until softened, about 5 minutes.
- Add crushed tomatoes, tomato paste, oregano, and basil. Bring to a simmer and cook for 10 minutes, stirring occasionally.
- Drain cooked spaghetti and return it to the pot.
- Add tomato sauce and parsley to the spaghetti and toss to combine.
- Season with salt and pepper to taste.
- Serve immediately.

6. **Baked Tofu with Roasted Vegetables:**

Ingredients:

- 1 (14-ounce) package extra-firm tofu, drained and pressed
- 1 tablespoon olive oil
- 1/2 teaspoon dried oregano
- 1/4 teaspoon salt
- 1/4 teaspoon black pepper
- 1 cup broccoli florets
- 1/2 cup red bell pepper, sliced

- 1/2 cup yellow bell pepper, sliced

- 1/2 cup red onion, sliced

Instructions:

- Preheat oven to 400°F (200°C).

- Cut tofu into cubes about 1 inch in size.

- In a bowl, toss tofu with olive oil, oregano, salt, and pepper.

- Arrange tofu cubes on a baking sheet lined with parchment paper.

- Toss broccoli, bell peppers, and onion with olive oil, salt, and pepper.

- Spread vegetables around the tofu on the baking sheet.

- Bake for 20-25 minutes, or until tofu is golden brown and vegetables are tender.

7. **One-Pan Lemon Chicken with Roasted Asparagus:**

Ingredients:

- 4 boneless, skinless chicken breasts

- 1 tablespoon olive oil

- 1/2 teaspoon dried thyme

- 1/4 teaspoon salt

- 1/4 teaspoon black pepper

- 1 pound asparagus, trimmed and cut into 2-inch pieces
- 1 lemon, sliced

Instructions:

- Preheat oven to 425°F (220°C).
- In a bowl, toss chicken with olive oil, thyme, salt, and pepper.
- Arrange chicken on a baking sheet lined with parchment paper.
- Surround chicken with asparagus and lemon slices.
- Roast for 20-25 minutes, or until chicken is cooked through and asparagus is tender-crisp

.

8.   **Shrimp Stir-Fry with Quinoa:**

Ingredients:

- 1 pound shrimp, peeled and deveined
- 1 tablespoon cornstarch
- 1 tablespoon soy sauce
- 1 tablespoon rice vinegar
- 1 tablespoon honey
- 1 tablespoon olive oil
- 1 onion, chopped
- 2 carrots, chopped

                     Pritkin Diet and Meal Plan

- 1 red bell pepper, chopped
- 1 cup cooked quinoa
- 1/4 cup chopped fresh cilantro
- Sesame seeds (optional)

Instructions:

- In a bowl, toss shrimp with cornstarch, soy sauce, rice vinegar, and honey.
- Heat olive oil in a large skillet or wok over medium-high heat.
- Add shrimp and cook until pink and cooked through, about 2-3 minutes per side.
- Remove shrimp from the pan and set aside.
- Add onion, carrots, and bell pepper to the pan and cook until softened, about 5 minutes.
- Stir in cooked quinoa and shrimp.
- Cook for 1 minute to heat through.
- Garnish with chopped cilantro and sesame seeds (optional).

9. Vegetarian Stuffed Peppers:

Ingredients:

- 4 bell peppers
- 1 cup brown rice, cooked

- 1 cup black beans, drained and rinsed
- 1 (10-ounce) can diced tomatoes with green chilies, undrained
- 1/2 cup chopped onion
- 1/4 cup chopped fresh cilantro
- 1 tablespoon chili powder
- 1 teaspoon cumin
- 1/2 teaspoon dried oregano
- 1/4 cup shredded cheese (optional)

Instructions:

- Preheat oven to 375°F (190°C).
- Cut the tops off the bell peppers and remove the seeds and membranes.
- In a large bowl, combine cooked brown rice, black beans, diced tomatoes with green chilies, onion, cilantro, chili powder, cumin, and oregano.
- Mix well.
- Fill each bell pepper with the rice mixture.
- Place the stuffed peppers in a baking dish.
- Bake for 30-35 minutes, or until bell peppers are tender and filling is heated through.
- Top with shredded cheese (optional) and serve immediately.

Ingredients:

- 1 tablespoon olive oil
- 1 onion, chopped
- 2 cloves garlic, minced
- 1 tablespoon curry powder
- 1 teaspoon ground turmeric
- 1/2 teaspoon ground cumin
- 1/4 teaspoon red pepper flakes (optional)
- 1 cup lentils, rinsed
- 4 cups vegetable broth
- 1 (14.5-ounce) can diced tomatoes, undrained
- 1 cup chopped fresh spinach
- Salt and pepper to taste
- Naan bread, for serving

Instructions:

- Heat olive oil in a large pot or Dutch oven over medium heat.
- Add onion and garlic, and cook until softened, about 5 minutes.

- Add curry powder, turmeric, cumin, and red pepper flakes (optional). Cook for 1 minute, stirring constantly.
- Stir in lentils, vegetable broth, and diced tomatoes with their juices.
- Bring to a boil, then reduce heat and simmer for 30 minutes, or until lentils are tender.
- Stir in spinach and cook until wilted, about 1 minute.
- Season with salt and pepper to taste.
- Serve hot with naan bread.

These 10 delicious and nutritious Pritikin dinner recipes offer a variety of flavors and textures to keep your evenings exciting and satisfying. Remember, dinner is a time to relax and unwind after a long day. Choose meals that are nourishing and enjoyable, and you'll be well on your way to a healthier and happier you.

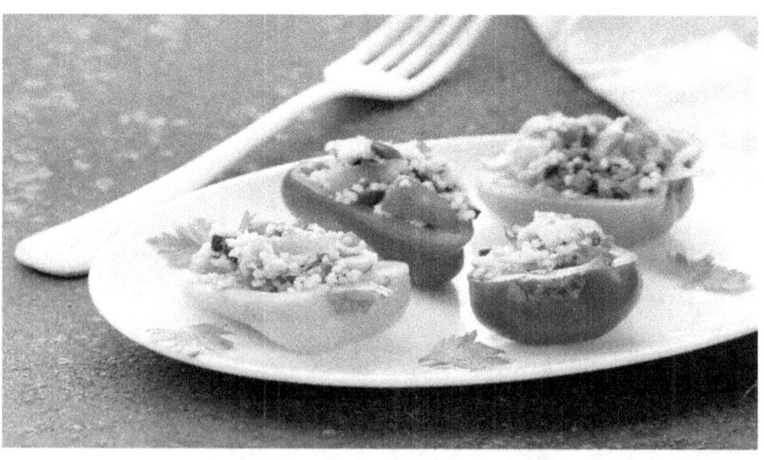

CHAPTER 5

SNACKS:

Nutritious and Satisfying Pritikin Snacks

It is important to keep your body energized through constant eating of healthy snacks between meals in order to avoid excessive eating at supper time. In chapter 5, there are 10 quick and healthy Pritikin snack ideas. They are delicious and will nourish you all through the day. These snacks include fruits and vegetables, nuts and seeds as well as creamy yoghurts, hard boiled eggs and whole-wheat crackers with low-fat cheese catering for all types of cravings and dietary preferences. We shall look at some delicious morsels that make your tongue smile and your body healthy.

1. **Fruits and Vegetables:**

Ingredients:

- Fresh fruits of your choice (e.g., apples, bananas, berries, grapes)
- Fresh vegetables of your choice (e.g., baby carrots, celery sticks, cucumber slices)

Instructions:

- Wash and prepare your chosen fruits and vegetables.

- Enjoy them plain or pair them with a small amount of natural nut butter for added protein and healthy fats.

2. **Nuts and Seeds:**

Ingredients:

- 1/4 cup almonds, walnuts, cashews, pecans, or a mix of your choice

- 1/4 cup pumpkin seeds, sunflower seeds, chia seeds, or flaxseeds

Instructions:

- Dry roast nuts and seeds in a pan for a few minutes to enhance their flavor.

- Enjoy them as a snack on their own or add them to yogurt, salads, or oatmeal for extra crunch and nutrition.

3. **Yogurt:**

Ingredients:

- 1 cup plain Greek yogurt

- 1/4 cup fresh or frozen berries

- 1 teaspoon honey or maple syrup (optional)
- 1/4 cup granola (optional)

Instructions:

- Mix plain Greek yogurt with your chosen berries and sweetener (if desired).
- Top with granola for added texture and fiber.

4. **Hard-Boiled Eggs:**

Ingredients:

- Eggs (quantity as desired)
- Water
- **Salt (optional)**

Instructions:

- Place eggs in a saucepan and cover with water.
- Bring to a boil, then remove from heat and cover.
- Let eggs sit for 12-15 minutes for hard-boiled yolks.
- Rinse eggs under cold water and peel.
- Season with salt to taste (optional).

5. **Whole-Wheat Crackers and Low-Fat Cheese:**

Ingredients:

- 10-15 whole-wheat crackers
- 2 slices low-fat cheddar cheese
- Sliced tomato or cucumber (optional)

Instructions:

- Arrange whole-wheat crackers on a plate.
- Top each cracker with a piece of low-fat cheese.
- Add sliced tomato or cucumber for additional flavor and nutrients (optional).

6. Trail Mix:

Ingredients:

- 1/4 cup mixed nuts and seeds
- 1/4 cup dried fruits (e.g., raisins, cranberries, apricots)
- 1/4 cup dark chocolate chips (optional)
- Instructions:
- Combine nuts and seeds of your choice with dried fruits.
- Add dark chocolate chips for a decadent touch (optional).
- Store in an airtight container and enjoy as a satisfying snack on the go.

Ingredients:

- 1 (15-ounce) can chickpeas, drained and rinsed
- 1 tablespoon olive oil
- 1/2 teaspoon cumin
- 1/4 teaspoon chili powder
- Salt and pepper to taste

Instructions:

- Preheat oven to 400°F (200°C).
- Toss drained chickpeas with olive oil, cumin, chili powder, salt, and pepper.
- Spread chickpeas on a baking sheet and roast for 20-25 minutes, or until crisp and golden brown.
- Enjoy these savory roasted chickpeas on their own or sprinkled over salads for a protein boost.

8.   Edamame:

Ingredients:

- 1 cup frozen edamame pods
- 1 tablespoon olive oil
- 1/4 teaspoon sea salt

Instructions:

- Thaw frozen edamame pods according to package instructions.
- Heat olive oil in a pan over medium heat.
- Add edamame pods and cook for 5-7 minutes, or until heated through.
- Sprinkle with sea salt and enjoy as a warm and flavorful snack.

9. Carrot Sticks with Hummus:

Ingredients:

- 2-3 large carrots, cut into sticks
- 1/4 cup homemade or store-bought hummus

Instructions:

- Wash and slice carrots into sticks for easy dipping.
- Enjoy the crunchy carrot sticks with creamy hummus for a satisfying and healthy snack.

10. Apple Slices with Almond Butter:

Ingredients:

- 1 apple, sliced

- 2 tablespoons natural almond butter

Instructions:

- Wash and slice the apple into thin slices.
- Spread almond butter on the apple slices for a delicious and protein-rich treat.

These 10 nutritious and satisfying Pritikin snack recipes offer a variety of flavors and textures to keep you energized and satisfied between meals. Remember, choosing healthy snacks can help you maintain a balanced diet and reach your health goals. So, ditch the processed snacks and explore the world of delicious and nutritious options presented in this chapter. Your body and taste buds will thank you for it!

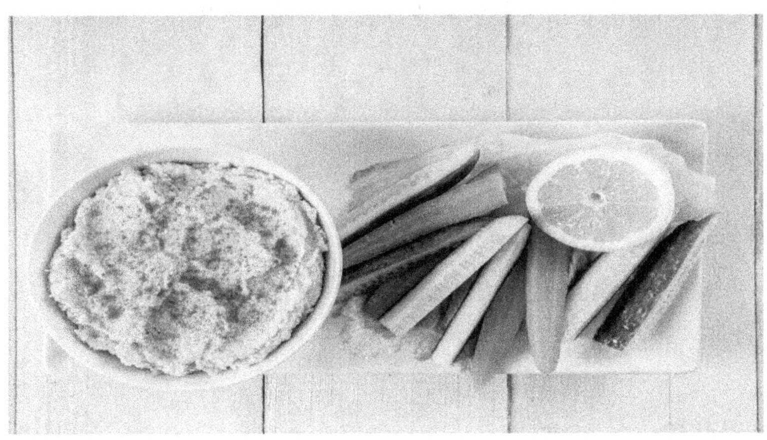

CHAPTER 6

DESSERTS:

Delicious and Healthy Pritikin Desserts

You don't have to deprive yourself of those sweets just because you want to achieve your fitness and health objectives. In chapter six you will find out how to make mouthwatering Pritikin desserts without harming you. This chapter discusses different types of sweet foods like fruity and refreshing frugal parfaits, creamy and decadent mousses and baked treats with a healthy touch. These desserts show that health can truly be delicious as a fresh palate to close off a meal or as an awesome dessert to share with loved ones.

1. Fruit Salad with Yogurt and Honey:

Ingredients:

- 1 cup mixed seasonal fruits (e.g., berries, melon, grapes)
- 1/2 cup plain Greek yogurt
- 1 tablespoon honey

Instructions:

- Combine your chosen fruits in a bowl.
- Top with plain Greek yogurt and drizzle with honey.

- Enjoy this light and refreshing dessert for a satisfying end to a meal.

2. **Dark Chocolate and Almond Bark:**

Ingredients:

- 1/2 cup dark chocolate chips (70% cacao or higher)
- 1/4 cup almonds, chopped

Instructions:

- Melt dark chocolate chips in a microwave-safe bowl according to package instructions.
- Stir in chopped almonds.
- Pour melted chocolate onto a baking sheet lined with parchment paper.
- Refrigerate for at least 30 minutes until hardened.
- Break the chocolate bark into pieces and enjoy this decadent and healthy treat.

3. **Frozen Banana Bites:**

Ingredients:

- 2 ripe bananas
- 1 tablespoon melted dark chocolate (optional)

- Toppings of your choice (e.g., chopped nuts, shredded coconut, granola)

Instructions:

- Peel and slice bananas into bite-sized pieces.
- Freeze banana slices for at least 2 hours until frozen solid.
- Dip frozen banana slices in melted dark chocolate (optional).
- Roll the dipped banana slices in your chosen toppings.
- Enjoy these refreshing and healthy frozen treats.

4. **Chia Pudding with Berries and Coconut:**

Ingredients:

- 1/4 cup chia seeds
- 1 cup unsweetened plant-based milk
- 1/4 cup fresh berries
- 1 tablespoon shredded coconut

Instructions:

- Combine chia seeds and plant-based milk in a jar.
- Stir well and refrigerate for at least 4 hours, or overnight for a thicker consistency.

- In the morning, top the chia pudding with fresh berries and shredded coconut.
- Enjoy this creamy and satisfying pudding for a healthy and delicious breakfast or snack.

5. **Baked Apples with Cinnamon and Raisins:**

Ingredients:

- 2 apples
- 1 teaspoon cinnamon
- 1/4 cup raisins
- 1 tablespoon water

Instructions:

- Preheat oven to 375°F (190°C).
- Core apples and place them in a baking dish.
- Combine cinnamon and raisins and fill the cored apples with this mixture.
- Add 1 tablespoon of water to the bottom of the baking dish.
- Bake apples for 30-35 minutes, or until tender.
- Enjoy these baked apples warm for a comforting and healthy dessert.

6. **Coconut Mango Mousse:**

Ingredients:

- 1 ripe mango, peeled and chopped
- 1 (13.5-ounce) can unsweetened coconut milk, chilled
- 1/4 cup agave nectar
- 1 teaspoon vanilla extract

Instructions:

- Blend together chopped mango, coconut milk, agave nectar, and vanilla extract until smooth.
- Pour the mousse into individual serving cups.
- Refrigerate for at least 2 hours until chilled and thickened.
- Enjoy this creamy and tropical mousse for a refreshing and healthy dessert.

7. **Roasted Pears with Honey and Ginger:**

Ingredients:

- 2 ripe pears
- 1 tablespoon honey
- 1/2 teaspoon ground ginger

Instructions:

- Preheat oven to 375°F (190°C).

                     Pritkin Diet and Meal Plan

- Core pears and cut th'em into halves.

- Drizzle pears with honey and sprinkle with ground ginger.

- Place pears on a baking sheet and roast for 20-25 minutes, or until tender.

- Enjoy these roasted pears warm for a simple and flavorful dessert.

8. **No-Bake Energy Bites:**

Ingredients:

- 1 cup rolled oats

- 1/2 cup chopped almonds

- 1/4 cup pitted dates

- 1/4 cup dried cranberries

- 1 tablespoon unsweetened cocoa powder

- 1 tablespoon coconut oil, melted

Instructions:

- In a food processor, pulse together rolled oats, almonds, dates, and cranberries until finely chopped.

- Add cocoa powder and melted coconut oil and process until combined.

- Roll the mixture into bite-sized balls.

- Refrigerate for at least 30 minutes until firm.

- Enjoy these no-bake energy bites for a quick and healthy snack or dessert.

9. **Baked Sweet Potato Fries with Cinnamon and Maple Syrup:**

Ingredients:

- 1 sweet potato
- 1 teaspoon cinnamon
- 1 tablespoon maple syrup
- 1 tablespoon olive oil

Instructions:

- Preheat oven to 400°F (200°C).
- Peel and cut the sweet potato into thin fries.
- Toss sweet potato fries with cinnamon, maple syrup, and olive oil.
- Spread fries on a baking sheet and bake for 20-25 minutes, or until golden brown and crispy.
- Enjoy these baked sweet potato fries for a healthier twist on a classic dessert.

10. **Chocolate Avocado Pudding:**

Ingredients:

- 1 ripe avocado
- 1/2 cup unsweetened cocoa powder
- 1/4 cup honey
- 1 teaspoon vanilla extract
- 1/4 cup milk (optional)

Instructions:

- Blend together avocado, cocoa powder, honey, vanilla extract, and milk (if desired) until smooth and creamy.
- Adjust the sweetness to your preference by adding more honey if needed.
- Serve this chocolate avocado pudding immediately for a rich and decadent dessert.

Remember, indulging in sweets can still be part of a healthy lifestyle when done thoughtfully. Choose desserts made with wholesome ingredients and enjoy them in moderation. This chapter provides a delicious way to satisfy your sweet tooth without compromising your health goals. So go ahead, explore and enjoy these healthy and satisfying Pritikin desserts!

SIDE DISHES:

Delicious and Nutritious Pritikin Side Dishes

Side dishes are usually unnoticed supermen of meal who add brightness, taste, and richness to the main course. However, they should not be pushed to the sidelines. Chapter 7 features 10 Pritikin-approved side dishes in order, all of which deserve their own chapter. With anything from vibrant roasted vegetables to hearty grilled corn on the cob, through refreshing salads to satisfying baked potatoes, these recipes provide plenty of choice to go with any meal. Thus throw the processed side dishes aside and consider trying these healthy and delicious alternatives that will have you craving for more.

1. Roasted Brussels Sprouts with Garlic and Herbs:

Ingredients:

- 1 pound Brussels sprouts, trimmed and halved
- 1 tablespoon olive oil
- 1/2 teaspoon garlic powder
- 1/4 teaspoon dried thyme

- Salt and pepper to taste

Instructions:

- Preheat oven to 400°F (200°C).
- Toss Brussels sprouts with olive oil, garlic powder, dried thyme, salt, and pepper.
- Spread Brussels sprouts on a baking sheet and roast for 20-25 minutes, or until tender and crispy.

2. **Grilled Corn on the Cob with Herbs:**

Ingredients:

- 4 ears of corn, husked
- 1 tablespoon olive oil
- 1/4 cup chopped fresh herbs (e.g., basil, cilantro, parsley)
- Salt and pepper to taste

Instructions:

- Preheat grill to medium heat.
- Brush corn with olive oil and season with salt and pepper.
- Grill corn for 15-20 minutes, turning occasionally, until tender and golden brown.
- Sprinkle grilled corn with chopped fresh herbs and serve.

3. **Quinoa Salad with Black Beans and Vegetables:**

 Pritkin Diet and Meal Plan

Ingredients:

- 1 cup cooked quinoa
- 1 (15-ounce) can black beans, drained and rinsed
- 1 cup chopped vegetables (e.g., red bell pepper, corn, cucumber)
- 1/4 cup chopped red onion
- 1/4 cup chopped fresh cilantro
- 2 tablespoons lime juice
- 1 tablespoon olive oil
- Salt and pepper to taste

Instructions:

- Combine cooked quinoa, black beans, chopped vegetables, red onion, and cilantro in a large bowl.
- Whisk together lime juice and olive oil to make a dressing.
- Pour dressing over the salad and toss to combine.
- Season with salt and pepper to taste.

4. Baked Potatoes with Herbs and Low-Fat Yogurt:

Ingredients:

- 2 large baking potatoes

- 1 tablespoon olive oil

- 1/2 teaspoon dried rosemary

- 1/4 cup low-fat plain yogurt

- Salt and pepper to taste

Instructions:

- Preheat oven to 400°F (200°C).

- Prick potatoes with a fork and rub with olive oil.

- Sprinkle with dried rosemary and salt.

- Bake potatoes for 45-60 minutes, or until tender.

- Top baked potatoes with low-fat yogurt and season with pepper to taste.

5. **Sautéed Green Beans with Garlic and Lemon:**

Ingredients:

- 1 pound fresh green beans, trimmed

- 1 tablespoon olive oil

- 2 cloves garlic, minced

- 1/4 cup lemon juice

- Salt and pepper to taste

Instructions:

- Heat olive oil in a large skillet over medium heat.

- Add green beans and cook for 5-7 minutes, or until tender-crisp.

- Add garlic and cook for 1 minute, stirring constantly.

- Stir in lemon juice and season with salt and pepper to taste.

- Serve immediately.

6. **Roasted Sweet Potato Wedges with Cinnamon and Cayenne Pepper:**

Ingredients:

- 1 large sweet potato

- 1 tablespoon olive oil

- 1/2 teaspoon cinnamon

- 1/4 teaspoon cayenne pepper (optional)

- Salt and pepper to taste

Instructions:

- Preheat oven to 425°F (220°C).

- Cut sweet potato into wedges.

- Toss wedges with olive oil, cinnamon, cayenne pepper (optional), salt, and pepper.

- Spread wedges on a baking sheet and roast for 20-25 minutes, flipping halfway through, until tender and golden brown.

7. **Steamed Broccoli with Lemon and Sesame Seeds:**

Ingredients:

- 1 head of broccoli, cut into florets
- 1 tablespoon lemon juice
- 1 tablespoon sesame seeds
- Salt and pepper to taste

Instructions:

- Steam broccoli florets for 5-7 minutes, or until tender-crisp.
- Drizzle with lemon juice and toss with sesame seeds.
- Season with salt and pepper to taste.

8. Grilled Portobello Mushrooms with Balsamic Glaze:

Ingredients:

- 2 large portobello mushrooms
- 1 tablespoon olive oil
- 1/4 cup balsamic vinegar
- 1 tablespoon honey
- Salt and pepper to taste

Instructions:

- Preheat grill to medium heat.

            Pritkin Diet and Meal Plan

- Brush portobello mushrooms with olive oil and season with salt and pepper.
- Grill mushrooms for 5-7 minutes per side, or until tender.
- Meanwhile, combine balsamic vinegar and honey in a saucepan and bring to a simmer.
- Reduce heat and simmer for 5-7 minutes, or until thickened.
- Brush grilled mushrooms with balsamic glaze and serve immediately.

9. **Roasted Asparagus with Herbs and Parmesan Cheese:**

Ingredients:

- 1 pound asparagus, trimmed
- 1 tablespoon olive oil
- 1/4 teaspoon dried oregano
- 1/4 cup grated Parmesan cheese (optional)
- Salt and pepper to taste

Instructions:

- Preheat oven to 400°F (200°C).
- Toss asparagus with olive oil, oregano, salt, and pepper.
- Spread asparagus on a baking sheet and roast for 10-12 minutes, or until tender-crisp.

- Sprinkle with grated Parmesan cheese (optional) and serve immediately.

Ingredients:

- 2 cups frozen edamame pods, thawed
- 1/4 teaspoon sea salt
- 1/4 teaspoon chili flakes (optional)

Instructions:

- Steam edamame pods for 5-7 minutes, or until heated through.
- Sprinkle with sea salt and chili flakes (optional).
- Serve immediately as a healthy and satisfying side dish.

Remember, side dishes are an opportunity to add variety and nutrition to your meals. Choose healthy ingredients and experiment with different flavors and textures to keep your meals exciting. This chapter provides a delicious and nutritious guide to elevate your mealtimes and nourish your body with every bite.

CHAPTER 8

SAUCES AND DIPS:

Flavorful and Healthy Pritikin Sauces and Dips

Every meal needs a finishing touch of sauce or dip that makes it even more delectable. However, most of the usual dips are loaded with unhealthy fats and salts making us feel guilty once we eat it. Pritikin Sauces is the chapter eight that delves into different healthy and flavorful sauces and dips which are friendly to health but still enhance your dietary intake. There is something for you whether you like creamy avocado dips, zesty salsas, refreshing yogurt sauces or herb-infused marinades. Get rid of those sauces you buy at the store, and try out some homemade ones that can please your palate and also benefit your health.

1. Avocado Cilantro Dip:

Ingredients:

- 1 ripe avocado
- 1/4 cup chopped fresh cilantro
- 2 tablespoons lime juice
- 1/4 teaspoon salt

- 1/8 teaspoon black pepper

Instructions:

- Mash the avocado in a bowl until smooth.
- Stir in chopped cilantro, lime juice, salt, and pepper.
- Serve this creamy and flavorful dip with vegetables, pita bread, or crackers.

2. Roasted Tomato Salsa:

Ingredients:

- 2 tomatoes, diced
- 1/2 red onion, diced
- 1/4 cup chopped fresh cilantro
- 2 tablespoons lime juice
- 1 tablespoon olive oil
- 1/2 teaspoon chili powder
- 1/4 teaspoon salt
- 1/8 teaspoon black pepper

Instructions:

- Preheat oven to 400°F (200°C).
- Toss diced tomatoes with olive oil, chili powder, salt, and pepper.

- Spread tomatoes on a baking sheet and roast for 15-20 minutes, or until softened and blistered.
- Combine roasted tomatoes with red onion, cilantro, lime juice, salt, and pepper.
- Serve this zesty and refreshing salsa with chips, tacos, or grilled meats.

3. Yogurt Dill Sauce:

Ingredients:

- 1 cup plain Greek yogurt
- 1/4 cup chopped fresh dill
- 1 tablespoon lemon juice
- 1/2 teaspoon garlic powder
- 1/4 teaspoon salt
- 1/8 teaspoon black pepper

Instructions:

- Combine all ingredients in a bowl and whisk until smooth.
- Serve this creamy and tangy yogurt sauce with roasted vegetables, grilled chicken, or fish.
-

4. Chimichurri Sauce:

Pritkin Diet and Meal Plan

Ingredients:

- 1/2 cup fresh parsley, chopped
- 1/4 cup fresh cilantro, chopped
- 2 cloves garlic, minced
- 1/4 cup olive oil
- 2 tablespoons red wine vinegar
- 1/2 teaspoon dried oregano
- 1/4 teaspoon salt
- 1/8 teaspoon black pepper

Instructions:

- Combine all ingredients in a food processor and pulse until finely chopped.
- Serve this flavorful chimichurri sauce with grilled meats, vegetables, or bread.

5. Lemon Garlic Marinade:

Ingredients:

- 1/4 cup olive oil
- 2 tablespoons lemon juice
- 1 tablespoon minced garlic
- 1/2 teaspoon dried oregano
- 1/4 teaspoon salt

          Pritkin Diet and Meal Plan

- 1/8 teaspoon black pepper

Instructions:

- Combine all ingredients in a bowl and whisk until well combined.
- Marinate your favorite protein (chicken, fish, tofu) in this flavorful mixture for at least 30 minutes or up to 24 hours for deeper flavor.

6. **Spicy Peanut Sauce:**

Ingredients:

- 1/2 cup natural peanut butter
- 1/4 cup low-sodium soy sauce
- 1/4 cup unsweetened rice vinegar
- 1 tablespoon honey
- 1 tablespoon sriracha (adjust amount for desired spice level)
- 1 clove garlic, minced
- 1/2 cup water

Instructions:

- Combine all ingredients in a blender and process until smooth.

　　Pritkin Diet and Meal Plan

- Thicken the sauce with additional water if necessary.

- Serve this spicy and flavorful peanut sauce with spring rolls, noodle dishes, or vegetables.

7.   Roasted Garlic Hummus:

Ingredients:

8.   1 (15-ounce) can chickpeas, drained and rinsed

9.   1/4 cup tahini

10. 2 tablespoons olive oil

11. 1 roasted garlic head, cloves squeezed out

12. 2 tablespoons lemon juice

13. 1/4 cup water

14. Salt and pepper to taste

Instructions:

- Combine all ingredients in a food processor and process until smooth and creamy.

- Adjust seasonings with salt and pepper to taste.

- Serve this delicious and healthy roasted garlic hummus with pita bread, vegetables, or crackers.

8.   Balsamic Vinaigrette:

Ingredients:

- 1/4 cup balsamic vinegar

- 2 tablespoons olive oil
- 1 tablespoon Dijon mustard
- 1/2 teaspoon dried oregano
- 1/4 teaspoon salt
- 1/8 teaspoon black pepperMB9999*9++999
- 9999

Instructions:

- Combine all ingredients in a jar and shake well to emulsify.
- Use this versatile balsamic vinaigrette to dress salads, marinate vegetables, or drizzle over grilled meats.

9. Creamy Herb Dressing:

Ingredients:

- 1/2 cup plain Greek yogurt
- 1/4 cup fresh herbs (e.g., dill, parsley, chives), chopped
- 1 tablespoon lemon juice
- 1/2 teaspoon Dijon mustard
- 1/4 teaspoon salt
- 1/8 teaspoon black pepper

Instructions:

- Combine all ingredients in a bowl and whisk until smooth.

- Use this creamy and flavorful herb dressing to dress salads, dip vegetables, or drizzle over grilled chicken or fish.

10. Mango Salsa with Mint:

Ingredients:

- 1 ripe mango, diced

- 1/2 red onion, diced

- 1/4 cup chopped fresh mint

- 2 tablespoons lime juice

- 1 tablespoon olive oil

- 1/2 teaspoon chili powder

- 1/4 teaspoon salt

- 1/8 teaspoon black pepper

Instructions:

- Combine all ingredients in a bowl and toss to coat.

- Serve this refreshing and flavorful mango salsa with chips, tacos, or grilled fish.

Remember, homemade sauces and dips offer a healthier and more flavorful alternative to store-bought options. Experiment with different ingredients and adjust seasonings to your liking to create your own signature dips and sauces. This chapter provides a delicious and nutritious guide to add a burst of flavor to your meals and enhance your dining experience. So, let your creativity flow and explore the world of homemade sauces and dips!

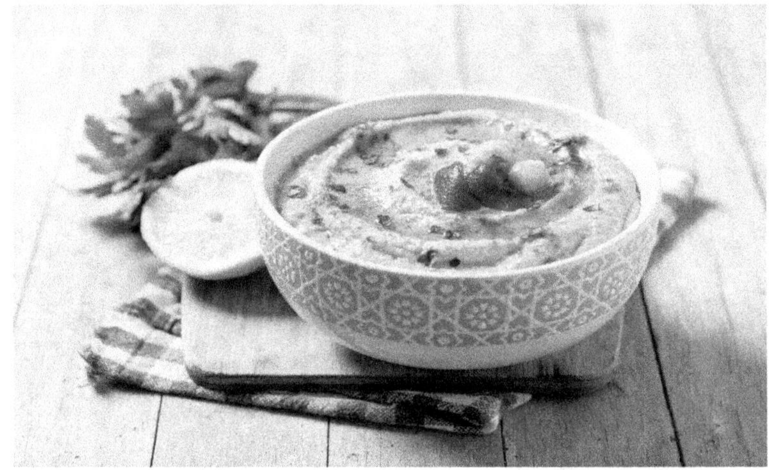

CHAPTER 9

MEAL PLANNING

Now you have a good fortune of delectable and healthful Pritikin recipes, it is time to put into practice. In chapter nine, it is all about meal planning, teaching you how to prepare nutritious and appetising food compatible with your schedule. Thus by observing the useful advice and techniques as given above, you will ensure that your refrigerator in the kitchen is well stocked with healthy foods and there are plans for meal time.

HOW TO CREATE A WEEKLY MEAL PLAN

Weekly meal planning is the best strategy a person can have if he/she wants to adopt a healthier lifestyle. The guesswork is removed when choosing a meal in a day, develops good eating habits, and saves time and money. Here's a comprehensive guide to help you create a weekly meal plan that works for you:

1.   **Set Your Goals and Preferences:**

Reflect on your goals: Do you want to lose weight, have more energy, address a specific health problem, or just eat better? Your food choices as well as meal planning decisions will be guided by identifying your goals.

- **Consider your preferences:** Are there any special nutritional requirements or food allergies? Are there any certain cuisines and meals that you prefer more? Consider your personal preferences in order for your meal plan to be sustainable as well as enjoyable.
- **Involve your family:** Discuss with your family what they desire and include them in planning. It fosters teamwork since every one has his or her favorite meal.

2.   Assess your Time and Resources:

Evaluate your schedule: Do you actually have enough time for cooking every day? Evaluate your working hours, errands and other commitments in order to determine how much time you are going to spend in the preparation of meals.

- **Determine your budget:** Determine a reasonable cost for groceries and prepare your meals as scheduled. Pay attention to what is in season and choose cheaper alternatives like legumes, whole grains, or frozen fruits and vegetables.

- **Utilize available resources:** Make time for preparing healthy food by considering strategies such as prepping ingredients, cooking in batches, and preserving leftovers. Get recipes and meal plan templates from blogs and online sources.

3. Plan your Meals:

- **Start with breakfast:** Choose healthy and satisfying breakfast options that provide sustained energy throughout the morning. Consider oatmeal with berries and nuts, yogurt with fruit and granola, or whole-wheat toast with avocado and eggs.

- **Move on to lunch and dinner:** Plan balanced meals that include whole grains, vegetables, lean protein, and healthy fats. Aim for variety and incorporate different cuisines and flavors to keep your meals exciting.

- **Don't forget snacks:** Plan healthy snacks to keep you energized throughout the day. Choose options like fruits and vegetables with nut butter, yogurt with granola, or whole-grain crackers with cheese.

4.   Create your Grocery List:

Review your meal plan: Make a list of all required food items for every meal and snack. Make sure that you stock up with basics such as olive oil, spices, and other condiments you would need.

- **Check your pantry and fridge**: Also, be sure to take stock of all your items so as to know everything that you already possess and do not repeat yourself while purchasing. It helps to save money and cut down on wastage of food.
- **Stick to your list:** Do not make a spur of the moment buying decision at the supermarket. Purchase only those things that are part of your list in order not to overspend and have unwise decisions.

5.   Prepare and Cook:

Dedicate time for meal prep: Pick one or two days per week and make meals ahead of time which can be divided into smaller portions. It is easy to do this during the week, as it saves time.

Get creative in the kitchen: Try out diverse cooking techniques like grilling, baking or even steaming so as to preserve the nutrient value and flavour of your foodstuffs.

Don't be afraid to ask for help: In case of limited time, meal delivery or requesting assistance from your friends will be beneficial in preparation or actual cooking.

6.   Adapt and Adjust:

Monitor your progress: At the end of the week, reflect on your weekly meal plan. Examine where you excelled and areas of improvement.

Be flexible: As required make alterations to your strategy. Sometimes you might need to diverge from the initial plan because of unexpected incidents or sudden change in preferences.

- **Embrace the journey:** Meal planning is an ongoing process of learning. Explore different recipes for healthful foods, while also having fun in creating these.

Remember, consistency is key. Practice makes perfect; the more you plan for meals the faster and smoother the process becomes. Incorporating these suggestions with adjustments to suit your specific demands will help you design a weekly menu that will take you towards a better and happier lifestyle.

One does not have to spend a lot of money when cooking nutritionally tasty foods. Planning and having some imagination will help you cook delicious dishes without spending much or eating too much. Practical tips and tricks on how to stretch your grocery budget will enable one to prepare tasty dishes, while still saving money.

PLANNING IS KEY:

- **Create a weekly meal plan:** It is a good idea to have planned your meals for the week in order not to make impulsive buys of things that are never needed at grocery stores.

- **Utilize grocery lists:** Ensure you stick to your shopping list and only buy what is on it to prevent impulsive purchases that can make a lot of difference in costs.

- **Take advantage of sales and coupons:** Cut coupons and create recipes using on-sale ingredients. Weekly flyers/online promotions are provided by many grocery stores.

- **Invest in pantry staples:** Keep your pantry stocked with multi-purpose items such as cereals, pasta, dried beans, vegetables in cans and jars, herbs and spices. They are

Pritkin Diet and Meal Plan

useful additions that can be incorporated into many dishes and form a base for healthy diets.

SMART SHOPPING STRATEGIES:

Compare prices: Comparing products unit prices in various supermarkets will be crucial for getting the best deal.

- **Buy in season:** More affordable seasonal produce may have a better taste.
- **Consider generic brands:** However, many generic brands provide similar quality as brand names but sell at low-cost prices.
- **Explore bulk options:** At the same time, buying some items in bulk as well, such as rice, bean or nut is cheaper than frequently acquiring small quantities of this kind of product..

Do not think of it that cooking on a budget means you have to forgo nutrition in terms of taste or nutrition. Hence, by adopting a creative approach to meal preparation, while still incorporating healthy and affordable choices, you can certainly prepare delicious and affordable meals that will suit your health needs. Therefore, cook creatively, enjoy being in the kitchen, and have the pleasure of the cheap cooking.

MEAL PLANNER

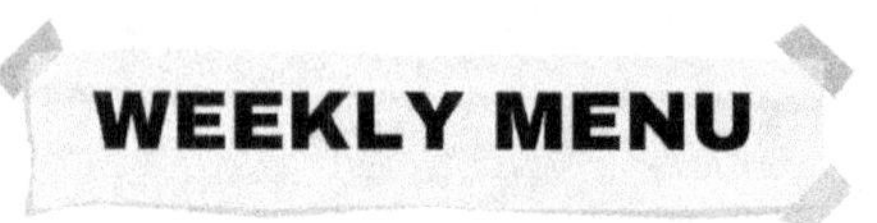

MONDAY

Breakfast:
Lunch:
Dinner:

TUESDAY

Breakfast:
Lunch:
Dinner:

WEDNESDAY

Breakfast:
Lunch:
Dinner:

THURSDAY

Breakfast:
Lunch:
Dinner:

FRIDAY

Breakfast:
Lunch:
Dinner:

SATURDAY

Breakfast:
Lunch:
Dinner:

SUNDAY

Breakfast:
Lunch:
Dinner:

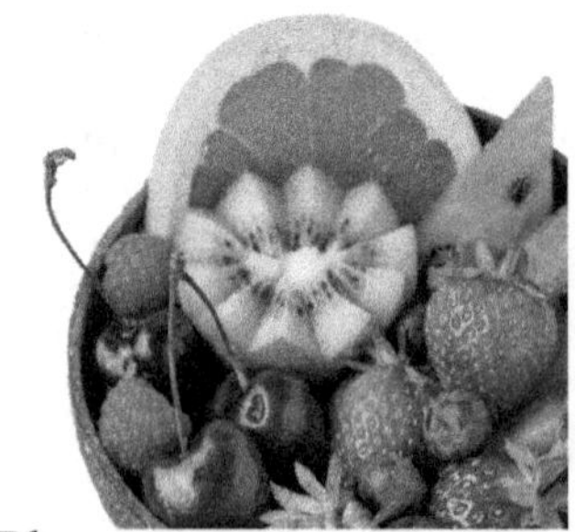

Pritkin Diet and Meal Plan

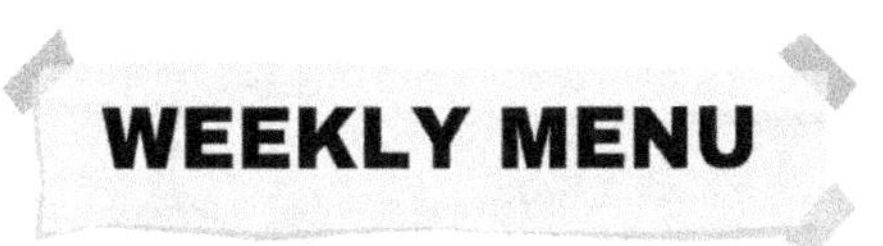

WEEKLY MENU

MONDAY

Breakfast:
Lunch:
Dinner:

FRIDAY

Breakfast:
Lunch:
Dinner:

TUESDAY

Breakfast:
Lunch:
Dinner:

SATURDAY

Breakfast:
Lunch:
Dinner:

WEDNESDAY

Breakfast:
Lunch:
Dinner:

SUNDAY

Breakfast:
Lunch:
Dinner:

THURSDAY

Breakfast:
Lunch:
Dinner:

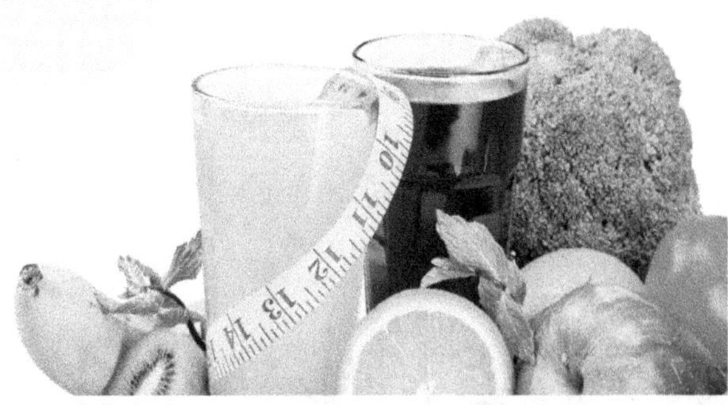

www.ingramcontent.com/pod-product-compliance
Lightning Source LLC
Chambersburg PA
CBHW060957260726
48661CB00005B/1909